This book was compiled by Daniel Melehi
with the A.I assistance of Inventabot

<u>Dedication</u>

I hope this helps all of my wonderful
readers achieve all their goals in their
business. And I would like to thank my
wonderful wife for all of her continued
support in all my ventures.

©Daniel Melehi

May 7 2023

Contents

Chapter 1: Introduction Behind the Unheard of Disease: Living with Wolfram Syndrome Welcome to Behind the Unheard of Disease: Living with Wolfram Syndrome. This book is intended to provide insight and support to those affected by Wolfram Syndrome, a rare genetic disorder that affects multiple systems in the body. Through personal stories and expert advice, this book aims to shed light on the challenges that individuals with Wolfram Syndrome and their families face and how to navigate them. As you read through the chapters of this book, you will gain a deeper understanding of Wolfram Syndrome, including its symptoms, diagnosis, and genetic inheritance. You will also learn about coping with the diagnosis and managing the condition, both through medical treatments and lifestyle adjustments. The emotional and psychological impacts of Wolfram

Syndrome will also be discussed, as well as relationships and hope for the future through current research and advocacy. Wolfram Syndrome is a complex and often difficult disease to manage, but this book is meant to serve as a guide and a source of inspiration. Whether you or someone you know has been affected by Wolfram Syndrome, this book offers a community of support and a reminder that you are not alone. So, let's begin this journey together, understanding and embracing the challenges of living with Wolfram Syndrome, and finding hope through knowledge and connection.

Behind the Unheard of Disease: Living with Wolfram Syndrome

Living with a rare disease can be overwhelming, isolating, and frustrating all at the same time. Wolfram Syndrome, also known as DIDMOAD, is one of the lesser-known genetic diseases that affect only a small number of people worldwide. It is a rare, neurodegenerative disorder that affects multiple body systems, including the eyes, central nervous system, and endocrine system. In this book, we will explore the experiences of people and families living with Wolfram Syndrome and provide insights on how they cope with the challenges associated with the disease. We will also delve into the current research on WS and how the medical community is working towards finding a cure for the disorder. Our hope is that this book will give you a better understanding of what it means to live with Wolfram Syndrome and help raise awareness about this rare disease. Join us as we embark on a journey to discover what it takes to live with a disease that many people have never heard of.

CHAPTER 1: INTRODUCTION

In this chapter, we will introduce you to Wolfram Syndrome, its causes, symptoms, and how it affects the lives of those who are diagnosed with the disorder. We will share stories of individuals living with WS, their families, and how they learned to navigate the challenges that come with it. You will also learn about the purpose of the book and what to expect in the upcoming chapters.

What is Wolfram Syndrome?

Wolfram Syndrome is a rare genetic disorder that affects various body systems, primarily the eyes, central nervous system, and endocrine system. Individuals diagnosed with Wolfram Syndrome experience progressive vision loss, diabetes insipidus, hearing loss, and neurodegenerative disorders, among other problems. The symptoms of the disease start appearing in early childhood, and in some cases, they may not be diagnosed until adulthood.

What Causes Wolfram Syndrome?

Wolfram Syndrome is caused by mutations in the WFS1 and CISD2 genes, which play a crucial role in regulating the production and secretion of insulin in the pancreas. The mutation of these genes leads to a decrease in the production of insulin, which results in diabetes insipidus and diabetes mellitus.

Living with Wolfram Syndrome

Living with Wolfram Syndrome is challenging, not only for the individuals who have been diagnosed with the disorder but also for their families. The physical and emotional toll of the disease can be overwhelming, and there is a lack of awareness and resources available to support patients and their families. In the upcoming chapters, we will explore how individuals with Wolfram Syndrome manage their symptoms, navigate healthcare, and seek support. We will also discuss the emotional impacts of the disease on individuals and their loved ones and what can be done to address them.

The Purpose of This Book

The primary purpose of this book is to provide insight into the experiences of individuals and families living with Wolfram Syndrome. We aim to raise awareness about this rare disease and provide support to those who are affected by it. Additionally, we will share current research and clinical trials and provide resources for advocacy and awareness for Wolfram Syndrome. We hope that through this book, we can empower individuals living with Wolfram Syndrome and their families by sharing their stories and insights into how to live a fulfilling life despite the challenges, and inspire the research and advocacy community to continue their work towards a cure. Thank you for joining us on this journey, and we hope you find this book informative, helpful, and inspiring.

Chapter 2: Understanding Wolfram Syndrome

Wolfram Syndrome, also known as DIDMOAD (diabetes insipidus, diabetes mellitus, optic atrophy, and deafness), is a rare genetic disorder that affects multiple parts of the body. This chapter aims to provide a deeper understanding of what Wolfram Syndrome is, its symptoms, and how it is diagnosed.

SUBCHAPTER 2.1: SYMPTOMS AND DIAGNOSIS

The symptoms of Wolfram Syndrome typically begin in childhood and manifest in several areas. Along with the four key symptoms of DIDMOAD - diabetes insipidus, diabetes mellitus, optic atrophy, and deafness, other symptoms may include bladder or bowel dysfunction, low muscle tone, mental health issues, and seizures. While not every individual diagnosed with

Wolfram Syndrome will exhibit all of these symptoms, many of these symptoms can occur as the condition progresses. Due to its rarity and the combination of multiple symptoms, Wolfram Syndrome can be difficult to diagnose. Typically, genetic testing is the most effective way to confirm a diagnosis. However, this can be a long and difficult process that can often lead to a misdiagnosis initially. It is essential that individuals who exhibit any of the hallmark symptoms of Wolfram Syndrome consult with a specialist as soon as possible.

SUBCHAPTER 2.2: GENETIC INHERITANCE

Wolfram Syndrome is caused by recessive mutation of the WFS1 gene, located on chromosome 4. This mutation is inherited in an autosomal recessive manner, meaning that an individual must inherit two copies of the mutated gene (one from each parent) to develop the condition. This results in a 25% chance of developing the condition with each child born to parents who both carry the mutation. It is also important to note that individuals with Wolfram Syndrome have a 50% chance of passing the mutation on to their children. For this reason, genetic counseling is essential for individuals with Wolfram Syndrome who are considering starting a family. Overall, understanding the symptoms and genetic inheritance of Wolfram Syndrome is essential for an accurate diagnosis and to a better quality of life for those affected by the condition.

SUBCHAPTER 2.1: SYMPTOMS AND DIAGNOSIS

Wolfram Syndrome is a rare genetic disease that affects multiple organs and systems in the body. While the symptoms can vary from person to person, there are several hallmark symptoms that are associated with this disease. One of the most common early symptoms of Wolfram Syndrome is vision loss, which can occur in childhood or adolescence. This vision loss is typically progressive and can lead to complete blindness in some cases. Patients may also experience optic nerve atrophy, which is the degeneration of the optic nerve that can result in a loss of peripheral vision. In addition to vision loss, many patients with Wolfram Syndrome also experience diabetes mellitus-type 1, which can develop in childhood or adolescence. This type of diabetes occurs when the body is unable to produce insulin, which can lead to high blood sugar levels and a range of complications. Other symptoms of Wolfram Syndrome can include hearing loss, bladder dysfunction, gastrointestinal issues, and neurological symptoms such as ataxia (loss of control over body movements) and seizures. Some patients also develop psychiatric symptoms such as depression, anxiety, and behavioral changes. Diagnosing Wolfram Syndrome can be challenging because of its rarity and variable presentation. However, certain diagnostic criteria have been established to help healthcare professionals identify the disease. These criteria include the presence of diabetes mellitus-type 1 and optic nerve atrophy, as well as at least one other symptom such as sensorineural hearing loss or neurological symptoms. Genetic testing can also be used to confirm a diagnosis of Wolfram Syndrome, as the disease is caused by mutations in the WFS1 gene. Genetic counseling is also recommended for patients and families affected by this disease. If you or someone you know is experiencing symptoms of Wolfram Syndrome, it is important to seek the guidance of a healthcare professional who is familiar with this rare disease. Early diagnosis and management of symptoms can improve outcomes and quality of life for patients and their families.

UNDERSTANDING WOLFRAM SYNDROME

Subchapter 2.2: Genetic Inheritance

Wolfram Syndrome, also known as DIDMOAD (Diabetes Insipidus, Diabetes Mellitus, Optic Atrophy, and Deafness), is a rare genetic disorder that affects around one in every 500,000 people. It is an autosomal recessive disorder, which means a person needs to inherit two copies of the defective gene (one from each parent) to develop the condition. The gene that causes Wolfram Syndrome is located on chromosome 4 and is called the WFS1 gene. The WFS1 gene encodes for the protein wolframin, which is involved in the regulation of calcium homeostasis, protecting cells from endoplasmic reticulum (ER) stress and beta-cell function. Mutations in the WFS1 gene affect the production or function of wolframin, leading to ER stress and cell death in various tissues, including the eyes, ears, brain, and endocrine pancreas. If both parents carry a single copy of the abnormal WFS1 gene, each of their children has:

- A 25% chance of inheriting both copies of the abnormal gene and developing Wolfram Syndrome
- A 50% chance of inheriting only one copy of the abnormal gene and becoming a carrier of the condition (with no symptoms)
- A 25% chance of inheriting both normal copies of the gene and not having the condition and not being a carrier

It is vital for families with a history of Wolfram Syndrome to undergo genetic testing to determine if they carry the abnormal WFS1 gene. Genetic counseling is also essential to discuss the inheritance pattern and the potential risks for their children. Being born with Wolfram Syndrome is not something anyone can control, and everyone deserves love, support, and understanding from their families and communities. In the following chapter, we will discuss how to cope with a Wolfram Syndrome diagnosis.

Chapter 3: Coping with Diagnosis

INTRODUCTION

Receiving a diagnosis of Wolfram Syndrome can be overwhelming and difficult for both the individual with the disease and their loved ones. It can be challenging to navigate the healthcare system, come to terms with the symptoms and impact on daily life, and find support during this time. In this chapter, we will discuss strategies for coping with a diagnosis of Wolfram Syndrome.

3.1 NAVIGATING HEALTHCARE

Receiving a diagnosis of Wolfram Syndrome can be a daunting and overwhelming experience for many families. It is important to remember that navigating the healthcare system effectively can help to alleviate some of the stress associated with a diagnosis. Some tips for navigating healthcare include:

Find a Specialist

One of the most important steps to navigating healthcare when living with Wolfram Syndrome is to find a healthcare specialist who is knowledgeable and experienced in treating the disease. It may be helpful to ask your primary care physician, or other healthcare providers for a recommendation. You can also reach out to support groups, advocacy organizations, and local hospitals for referrals.

Build a Healthcare Team

In addition to finding a specialist, it is important to build a team of healthcare providers that can help to manage other symptoms and conditions that may arise as a result of Wolfram Syndrome. This may include a mental health provider, physical therapist, ophthalmologist, and neurologist, among other specialists.

Stay Organized

Managing healthcare appointments, medications, and other important information can be challenging. It may be helpful to use a notebook, planner, or digital tool to keep track of appointments, medications, and any changes in symptoms or condition.

3.2 SUPPORT SYSTEMS

Coping with a diagnosis of Wolfram Syndrome can be an emotionally and physically taxing experience. It is important to build a strong support system to help manage these challenges. Here are some strategies for building a support system:

Connect with Other Families

Support groups, advocacy organizations, and social media groups can be valuable resources for connecting with other families affected by Wolfram Syndrome. These groups can provide emotional support, helpful resources, and information about coping strategies.

Lean on Family and Friends

Family and friends can also be important sources of support during this time. It may be helpful to have regular check-ins or gatherings with loved ones to talk about any challenges or concerns related to the disease.

Seek Mental Health Support

Living with Wolfram Syndrome can take a toll on mental health. Seeking the help of a mental health provider, such as a therapist or counselor, can be beneficial for managing anxiety, depression, and other mental health challenges.

CONCLUSION

Coping with a diagnosis of Wolfram Syndrome can be challenging, but there are many strategies for managing the emotional and logistical challenges that come with it. Navigating the healthcare system effectively, building a strong support system, and seeking mental health support are all important steps that can help individuals and families affected by Wolfram Syndrome manage the disease and maintain a high quality of life.

CHAPTER 3: COPING WITH DIAGNOSIS

Subchapter 3.1: Navigating Healthcare

Receiving a diagnosis of Wolfram Syndrome can be a difficult and overwhelming experience. Once the initial shock wears off, it's important to begin navigating the healthcare system in order to effectively manage the disease. Here are some tips to help you start: **Find a Specialist:** The first step in managing Wolfram Syndrome is finding a healthcare provider who specializes in rare genetic diseases. These specialists can offer valuable guidance on how to manage the disease and provide access to the most up-to-date treatments. **Understand Your Insurance Coverage:** Wolfram Syndrome requires lifelong management, and the cost of care can be quite high. It is important to understand your insurance coverage, including what is covered and what is not, in order to make informed decisions about your care. **Keep Detailed Records:** Keeping track of appointments, medications, and test results can help you stay organized and ensure that nothing falls through the cracks. This can also be helpful if you need to switch healthcare providers or seek a second opinion. **Communicate with Your Healthcare Team:** It is important to establish good communication with your healthcare team, including your doctor, nurse, and any other specialists you may be seeing. Keeping them informed of any changes in your symptoms or concerns can help ensure that you are receiving the best possible care. Remember, managing Wolfram Syndrome is a team effort, and you are an important part of that team. By taking an active role in your healthcare, you can help ensure the best possible outcome for yourself or your loved one.

SUBCHAPTER 3.2: SUPPORT SYSTEMS

Living with Wolfram Syndrome can be a challenging experience, not just for the affected individual, but for their loved ones as well. Therefore, it is essential to build a strong support system to help you or your loved one manage this condition better. One of the primary support systems for individuals with Wolfram Syndrome is family members. They provide emotional support, assist with daily tasks and help make important decisions regarding medical care. Additionally, family members can help ensure that the individual is adhering to their treatment plan and can provide caregivers with a break when needed. Another form of support is peer support. Advocacy networks, such as The Wolfram Syndrome UK Trust, offer peer support to individuals with Wolfram Syndrome and their families. They organize support group meetings where individuals can connect with others who have the same experiences. Peer support can be an excellent way for individuals and their families to share their experiences, ask questions, offer advice, and provide emotional support to one another. Community support is a key support system for individuals with Wolfram Syndrome. Local organizations and community groups can provide support in many different ways. This could involve fundraising for research or supporting individuals with Wolfram Syndrome to participate in community events. Additionally, local organizations can raise awareness and educate the community about Wolfram Syndrome, promoting acceptance and understanding. Finally, healthcare professionals can provide critical support to individuals with Wolfram Syndrome and their families. Healthcare providers, such as primary care physicians and specialists, not only diagnose and manage medical issues but can also offer counseling and connect individuals with other relevant healthcare professionals. They can help individuals navigate complex medical systems and ensure that they receive the care and support they need. In conclusion, having a strong support system is crucial for individuals with Wolfram Syndrome and their loved ones. Whether it is through family members, peer support, community groups, or healthcare professionals, support systems can provide critical emotional and practical support in managing this condition.

Chapter 4: Managing Wolfram Syndrome

Wolfram Syndrome is a rare and progressive disease that affects several systems of the body. Currently, there is no cure for Wolfram Syndrome, but there are several medical treatments and lifestyle adjustments that can help manage the symptoms of the disease.

SUBCHAPTER 4.1: MEDICAL TREATMENTS

While there is no cure for Wolfram Syndrome, there are several medical treatments that can help manage the disease. These treatments mainly focus on managing the symptoms and slowing the progression of the disease. One of the most common medical treatments for Wolfram Syndrome is insulin therapy. As the disease progresses, the pancreas becomes less and less effective at producing insulin, which can lead to high blood sugar levels. Insulin therapy involves injecting insulin into the body to help regulate blood sugar levels. Another common medical treatment for Wolfram Syndrome is hormone replacement therapy. As the disease progresses, the body may stop producing certain hormones, such as the hormones that regulate growth and development. Hormone replacement therapy involves taking synthetic versions of these hormones to help maintain healthy levels in the body. There are also several other medical treatments that may be used to manage the symptoms of Wolfram Syndrome, depending on the individual's specific symptoms and needs. These may include medications to manage bladder and bowel issues, as well as medications to manage the symptoms of depression and anxiety.

SUBCHAPTER 4.2: LIFESTYLE ADJUSTMENTS

In addition to medical treatments, there are also several lifestyle adjustments that can help manage the symptoms of Wolfram Syndrome. One of the most important lifestyle adjustments for individuals with Wolfram Syndrome is maintaining a healthy diet and exercise routine. Eating a balanced and healthy diet can help regulate blood sugar levels and maintain overall health, while regular exercise can help improve physical strength and alleviate symptoms such as muscle weakness. Another important lifestyle adjustment for individuals with Wolfram Syndrome is managing stress levels. Stress can exacerbate symptoms such as depression and anxiety, so finding healthy ways to manage stress, such as meditation or therapy, is crucial. Finally, it is important for individuals with Wolfram Syndrome to maintain regular check-ups with their healthcare provider. Monitoring the progression of the disease and any changes in symptoms is crucial for managing the disease effectively. In conclusion, while managing Wolfram Syndrome can be challenging, there are several medical treatments and lifestyle adjustments that can help manage symptoms and slow the progression of the disease. It is important for individuals with the disease to work closely with their healthcare team and maintain healthy habits in order to manage the disease as effectively as possible.

CHAPTER 4: MANAGING WOLFRAM SYNDROME

Subchapter 4.1: Medical Treatments

At present, there is no cure for Wolfram Syndrome, and treatment primarily focuses on managing the symptoms through targeted medical interventions. The treatment plan for each individual with

Wolfram Syndrome will vary depending on their unique set of symptoms. A team of healthcare professionals, including endocrinologists, ophthalmologists, audiologists, and neurologists, may coordinate to develop and implement a treatment plan. One of the primary symptoms of Wolfram Syndrome is diabetes insipidus, which can cause excessive thirst and urination. Treatment for this symptom usually involves desmopressin, a medication that stimulates the kidneys to retain water and reduce urine output. Another primary Symptom of Wolfram Syndrome is Diabetes mellitus, which is managed with insulin therapy. This treatment plan may involve daily injections of insulin or a continuous insulin infusion through an insulin pump. Blood glucose levels should be monitored regularly to avoid hypoglycemia or hyperglycemia. Wolfram Syndrome can also cause optic nerve atrophy, which can lead to vision loss. Treatments for this symptom may include correction with eyeglasses, contact lenses, or visual aids, such as magnifying glasses. Additionally, medications such as memantine, idebenone, or brimonidine, may be prescribed to help slow down the progression of optic nerve damage. Hearing loss is another common symptom of Wolfram Syndrome. Various hearing aids or cochlear implants may be used to treat this symptom. In some cases, other medications such as steroids may also be used to prevent further hearing loss. Lastly, neurological symptoms such as ataxia or tremors may be treated with medications that affect the central nervous system. Physical therapy can also help manage and improve motor coordination. In summary, there is no cure for Wolfram Syndrome, but targeted medical interventions can help manage symptoms related to diabetes insipidus, diabetes mellitus, optic nerve atrophy, hearing loss, and neurological symptoms. Treatment plans for each individual will vary depending on their unique set of symptoms, and it is important to work closely with healthcare professionals to develop and implement an effective treatment plan.

SUBCHAPTER 4.2: LIFESTYLE ADJUSTMENTS

Living with Wolfram Syndrome requires certain lifestyle changes to manage symptoms and improve overall health. Here are some lifestyle adjustments that individuals with Wolfram Syndrome or their caregivers can make:

Dietary Changes

A well-balanced, nutritious diet can improve overall health and reduce symptoms of Wolfram Syndrome. Individuals with Wolfram Syndrome are prone to diabetes, which means sugar intake needs to be monitored closely. A diet that emphasizes whole grains, fruits, vegetables, and lean protein can help manage blood sugar levels.

Physical Activity

Physical activity is vital for maintaining good health and reducing the risk of complications associated with Wolfram Syndrome. Exercise can help manage weight, improve blood sugar control, and reduce the risk of heart disease. It is essential to work with your healthcare team to develop a safe exercise plan that suits your individual needs and abilities.

Sleep

Getting an adequate amount of quality sleep is essential for overall health and wellness. Individuals with Wolfram Syndrome may experience sleep disturbances, which can impact their physical and mental health. It is essential to establish a regular sleep schedule and practice good sleep hygiene to promote restful sleep.

Stress Management

Living with a chronic illness can be stressful, and stress can exacerbate the symptoms of Wolfram Syndrome. It is crucial to develop effective coping mechanisms to manage stress, such as practicing relaxation techniques, seeking support from friends and family, and pursuing enjoyable activities.

Preventive Care

Regular check-ups and screenings are essential for preventing complications associated with Wolfram Syndrome. It is essential to work closely with your healthcare team to develop a preventive care plan that includes regular eye exams, kidney function tests, and hearing tests. By making these lifestyle adjustments, individuals with Wolfram Syndrome can effectively manage symptoms and improve their overall health. However, it is crucial to work closely with a healthcare team to develop an individualized plan that suits your unique needs and abilities.

Chapter 5: Wolfram Syndrome and Mental Health

Living with Wolfram Syndrome can be a challenging experience for those affected and their families. Apart from the physical symptoms, it can also take a toll on one's mental health. In this chapter, we will explore the emotional impacts of Wolfram Syndrome and how to seek professional help.

SUBCHAPTER 5.1: EMOTIONAL IMPACTS

The emotional impacts of Wolfram Syndrome are not just limited to those with the condition, but also to their family members and caregivers. Wolfram Syndrome is a progressive disease, which means that symptoms gradually worsen over time. Coping with the diagnosis and the uncertainty of how the disease will progress can be overwhelming and stressful. Some of the common emotional impacts of Wolfram Syndrome include:

Frustration and Anger

People living with Wolfram Syndrome may experience frustration and anger due to the limitations imposed by the condition. Simple everyday activities such as walking, eating, and communicating can become difficult or impossible, leading to feelings of frustration and anger.

Sadness and Depression

Prolonged feelings of sadness and depression are common amongst people living with Wolfram Syndrome. This may be due to the loss of independence and changes to the lifestyle or social life.

Anxiety and Fear

The uncertainty of the future and the progression of the disease can cause anxiety and fear. This can lead to problems with sleeping, eating, and other bodily functions.

SUBCHAPTER 5.2: SEEKING PROFESSIONAL HELP

Seeking professional help is crucial in managing the emotional impacts of Wolfram Syndrome. This can include therapy, medication, and support groups.

Therapy

Therapy can be helpful in developing coping mechanisms, managing stress, and improving communication skills. There are many different types of therapy available, including cognitive-behavioral therapy, talk therapy, and family therapy.

Medication

Antidepressants and anti-anxiety medication can help in managing the symptoms of depression and anxiety. It is important to consult with a healthcare professional before starting any medication.

Support Groups

Joining a support group can provide a sense of community, validation, and support. It can be beneficial to connect with people who are going through similar experiences and learn from their coping strategies.

CONCLUSION

Living with Wolfram Syndrome can be emotionally taxing for everyone involved. Recognizing the emotional impacts of the condition and seeking professional help can assist in managing these emotions. It is essential to focus on emotional health in addition to physical health when living with Wolfram Syndrome. Let's take care of ourselves and each other.

SUBCHAPTER 5.1: EMOTIONAL IMPACTS

Being diagnosed with Wolfram Syndrome can take a significant emotional toll on individuals affected by the disease, as well as their loved ones. In addition to the physical symptoms and complications associated with the disease, it can be challenging to cope with the psychological impact of Wolfram Syndrome. One of the significant emotional impacts of Wolfram Syndrome is the feeling of isolation and loneliness. Individuals with Wolfram Syndrome often feel cut off from their peers due to the rarity of the disease. They may feel that they are the only ones going through the experience, which can be daunting and overwhelming. Wolfram Syndrome can also cause anxiety, fear, and depression. Fear and anxiety are common when faced with the unknown. The future can be uncertain, and there is not enough information available on the prognosis of

Wolfram Syndrome. This uncertainty can lead to anxiety, which can sometimes become chronic. Depression is also common in individuals with Wolfram Syndrome. It is normal to feel sadness and grief when diagnosed with a chronic illness. However, depression is different from feeling sad. Depression is a long-lasting feeling of sadness, hopelessness, and helplessness. If left untreated, it can sometimes lead to suicidal thoughts. It is essential to consider and manage the psychological impact of Wolfram Syndrome on individuals with the disease. Seeking help from professionals, such as psychologists and psychiatrists, can be beneficial in dealing with the emotional and mental impacts of the disease. Support groups for individuals with Wolfram Syndrome and their families can also be helpful in connecting with others who understand the challenges. Overall, the emotional impacts of Wolfram Syndrome are significant. It is crucial to recognize the emotional toll that the disease can take on individuals and their loved ones and to seek support to manage these challenges.

SUBCHAPTER 5.2: SEEKING PROFESSIONAL HELP

Living with Wolfram Syndrome can be challenging, and it's essential to seek professional help to manage the mental health aspects of the disease. The emotional impacts of Wolfram Syndrome can be overwhelming, and it's not always easy to cope with them alone. This is where professional help comes into play. There are various mental health professionals available who can help you cope with the emotional impacts of Wolfram Syndrome. Some of the specialists you may encounter include psychologists, licensed clinical social workers, psychiatrists, and counselors. These professionals are trained to provide emotional support and guidance to those living with chronic diseases such as Wolfram Syndrome. When seeking professional help, it's essential to find someone who understands the unique challenges of living with a chronic illness such as Wolfram Syndrome. You may want to look for a mental health specialist who has experience working with individuals with chronic illnesses or disabilities. It's also crucial to find someone who makes you feel comfortable, supported, and understood. Therapy can be an effective way to address mental health concerns related to Wolfram Syndrome. Therapy gives you a safe and confidential space to discuss your feelings, thoughts, and experiences. This can help you process your emotions and develop coping strategies that work for you. Psychiatric medication is another option for individuals who are struggling with mental health aspects of Wolfram Syndrome. Antidepressants, anti-anxiety medications, and other psychiatric medications can help manage symptoms such as anxiety, depression, and mood swings. Your doctor can work with you to determine if medication is appropriate for your needs. In conclusion, seeking professional help is an essential step in managing the emotional impacts of Wolfram Syndrome. Whether you opt for therapy or medication, there are resources available to help you cope with the challenges of living with this disease. Don't hesitate to reach out for help if you're struggling – there is no shame in seeking help to take control of your mental and emotional well-being.

Chapter 6: Wolfram Syndrome and Relationships

Wolfram Syndrome not only affects the individual, but it can also have an impact on their relationships. Relationships can be challenging to navigate when dealing with a chronic disease like Wolfram Syndrome. In this chapter, we will explore the impact that Wolfram Syndrome can have on both familial and romantic relationships.

SUBCHAPTER 6.1: FAMILIAL RELATIONSHIPS

Families often play a significant supportive role in the lives of individuals with Wolfram Syndrome. As such, familial relationships can be both a source of comfort and a source of stress. The diagnosis of Wolfram Syndrome can be overwhelming for family members, particularly parents, who may experience feelings of guilt or helplessness. It is common for parents to want to help in any way possible, but they may not know how to do so. One of the best ways for family members to support their loved one with Wolfram Syndrome is by educating themselves on the disease. This includes understanding the symptoms, treatments, and progress of the disease. It is also important for family members to listen and communicate openly with their loved one. This can help keep communication lines open and support the person with Wolfram Syndrome. Families can also support their loved one with Wolfram Syndrome by creating a supportive environment that accommodates their needs. Adjustments to living spaces and routines can help individuals with Wolfram Syndrome live a more comfortable life. It is important for family members to work with their loved one to determine what adjustments are necessary and how they can be implemented.

SUBCHAPTER 6.2: ROMANTIC RELATIONSHIPS

The impact of Wolfram Syndrome on romantic relationships can be complex. For individuals with Wolfram Syndrome, dating can be challenging due to the impact of the disease on their daily routine and mental health. Relationships can also be affected by the progression of the disease. Communication is key in any relationship, but it is particularly important when a chronic disease is involved. It is important for individuals with Wolfram Syndrome to be open and honest with their partners about their condition and how it affects their daily life. This may include discussing adjustments that need to be made to accommodate their needs, such as scheduling dates earlier in the day or avoiding activities that may exacerbate their symptoms. Romantic partners can also be a great source of support for individuals with Wolfram Syndrome. Partners can offer emotional support and help with daily tasks or appointments. However, it is important to maintain a balance between supporting the person with Wolfram Syndrome and respecting their independence. In conclusion, relationships can be challenging to navigate when dealing with a chronic disease like Wolfram Syndrome. However, with education, communication, and support, both familial and romantic relationships can be strengthened. It is important for individuals with Wolfram Syndrome and their loved ones to work together to create a supportive environment that accommodates their needs and fosters strong relationships.

SUBCHAPTER 6.1: FAMILIAL RELATIONSHIPS

Wolfram Syndrome is a rare condition that affects not only the person diagnosed but also their family. It is important to understand how this syndrome can alter the dynamics of familial relationships and how to cope with such changes. Once a child is diagnosed with Wolfram Syndrome, the family must come to terms with the fact that life will be different. This can put a strain on relationships within the family, and extra effort may be required to maintain them. Parents may feel guilty and blame themselves for passing on the gene that caused the syndrome. Siblings may feel neglected as parents devote time and attention to the child with Wolfram Syndrome. One of the most challenging aspects of familial relationships with Wolfram Syndrome is the caregiving required. Individuals with Wolfram Syndrome often need assistance with daily activities, such as bathing, dressing, and eating. This responsibility often falls on the parents or siblings, which can result in emotional and physical exhaustion. It is crucial for caregivers to take care of their own well-being so they can offer the best possible care to their loved one. Communication is key in maintaining a healthy familial relationship. It is essential to keep channels of communication open and honest. Family members should express their feelings and concerns, including any frustrations, fears, or sadness. This can be accomplished through family meetings or individual conversations. When family members share what they are going through, they can better understand and empathize with each other, fostering a stronger bond. It is also important to seek outside support from friends, family, or professionals. Participating in support groups can be helpful for caregivers to share experiences and receive advice from others in similar situations. Therapists or counselors can also provide support and help family members process complicated emotions. In summary, familial relationships are significantly impacted by Wolfram Syndrome. Caregiving responsibilities and emotional stress can create difficulties within the family. However, by maintaining open and honest communication and seeking outside support, families can navigate these challenges together and grow stronger as a result.

CHAPTER 6.2: ROMANTIC RELATIONSHIPS

Living with Wolfram Syndrome can be challenging, not only for the individual with the condition, but also for their loved ones. Romantic relationships, in particular, can be affected by Wolfram Syndrome. In this subchapter, we will explore some of the challenges that individuals with Wolfram Syndrome may face in their romantic relationships and offer some tips for navigating these challenges.

The Challenges

Individuals with Wolfram Syndrome may face a variety of challenges in their romantic relationships. Some of these challenges may include:

- **Communication:** Individuals with Wolfram Syndrome may have difficulty communicating with their partner due to vision and hearing loss. It is important to find alternative methods for communication, such as using sign language or writing things down.
- **Physical Limitations:** Wolfram Syndrome can cause physical limitations, such as mobility issues. This may limit the activities that an individual with Wolfram Syndrome can do with their partner and may require some accommodations.
- **Emotional Challenges:** Wolfram Syndrome can cause emotional challenges such as depression and

anxiety, which can impact the individual's romantic relationship.

Navigating the Challenges

While the challenges of Wolfram Syndrome may seem daunting, there are ways to navigate them in order to maintain a healthy relationship. Here are some tips for navigating the challenges of romantic relationships with Wolfram Syndrome:

- **Open Communication:** It is important to maintain open communication with your partner. Discuss your needs and limitations and find ways to work around them together.
- **Adapt Activities:** If physical limitations are preventing you from doing certain activities, consider adapting them to make them more accessible. For example, if you enjoy hiking but have mobility issues, try hiking on more level terrain or using hiking poles for support.
- **Take Care of Your Mental Health:** Wolfram Syndrome can be emotionally challenging, so it is

important to take care of your mental health. This may involve seeking therapy or counseling to help manage feelings of depression and anxiety.

Conclusion

Romantic relationships can be challenging for anyone, but individuals with Wolfram Syndrome may face additional challenges. However, with open communication, adaptation, and prioritizing mental health, individuals with Wolfram Syndrome can navigate these challenges and maintain healthy romantic relationships.

Chapter 7: Hope for the Future

Living with Wolfram Syndrome can be challenging, but there is hope for the future. Advances in medical research and clinical trials are giving patients and their families new reasons to be optimistic.

SUBCHAPTER 7.1: CURRENT RESEARCH AND CLINICAL TRIALS

Researchers are actively searching for ways to improve the lives of those with Wolfram Syndrome. One promising avenue of research is the use of gene therapy. This approach involves correcting or replacing the faulty gene responsible for the disease. While still in the developmental stages, initial studies have shown promising results in treating related genetic diseases. Another area of research focuses on identifying biomarkers that could aid in early diagnosis and treatment. By tracking common markers of the disease, healthcare providers could intervene earlier and potentially delay symptoms. Clinical trials are another promising avenue for finding new treatments for Wolfram Syndrome. These trials aim to test the safety and effectiveness of new treatments and therapies. Many of these trials are focused on improving the management of symptoms and slowing the progression of the disease. Participating in a clinical trial can be a way to access new treatments that are not yet available to the general public.

SUBCHAPTER 7.2: ADVOCACY AND AWARENESS

Advocacy and awareness are critical components in advancing research and finding new treatments for Wolfram Syndrome. By raising awareness of the disease, we can increase funding for research and attract more researchers to the field. Advocacy can also bring greater attention to the difficulties faced by those living with the disease and their families. There are several organizations dedicated to advocacy and awareness for Wolfram Syndrome. The Diabetes Research Institute Foundation has established the Wolfram Syndrome International Registry and Clinical Study Group to help connect patients and researchers. Other organizations, such as the Snow Foundation and the Ellie White Foundation for Rare Genetic Disorders, also work to support research and raise awareness of the disease. In conclusion, while living with Wolfram Syndrome can be difficult, there is cause for hope. Advances in research and clinical trials are promising signs for the future. Advocacy and awareness can also play a crucial role in advancing research and improving the lives of those with the disease.

SUBCHAPTER 7.1: CURRENT RESEARCH AND CLINICAL TRIALS

Wolfram syndrome is a rare genetic disorder, and as such, research is limited. However, in recent years, there have been advances in understanding the disease, and efforts have been made towards finding treatment options. One of the focuses of research is on identifying the specific genes responsible for causing Wolfram syndrome.

This is crucial in preventing the disease from being passed down from generation to generation. Researchers have identified the WFS1 gene as one of the genes responsible for causing the disorder. However, there may be other genes involved, and further studies are being conducted to identify them. In addition to identifying the responsible genes, research is also being done to develop treatments for Wolfram syndrome. One promising area of research involves using gene therapy to correct the genetic abnormalities responsible for causing the disease. This involves replacing or modifying defective genes with normal, healthy ones. Clinical trials on the safety and efficacy of gene therapy are currently underway. Another area of research involves finding ways to prevent or slow down the progression of Wolfram syndrome. One drug that has shown promise in clinical studies is dantrolene, a medication commonly used to treat muscle spasms. Researchers think dantrolene may help protect the beta cells in the pancreas, which produce insulin and are typically destroyed in Wolfram syndrome. Finally, efforts are being made to improve supportive care for those with Wolfram syndrome. This includes developing better assistive technology to help with vision and hearing loss, as well as providing mental health support resources. In summary, while research on Wolfram syndrome is limited, there are promising areas of study aimed at identifying the responsible genes and developing treatments. Clinical trials are currently underway to determine the safety and effectiveness of these treatments. While there is still much to learn about this rare disease, the future looks hopeful.

SUBCHAPTER 7.2: ADVOCACY AND AWARENESS

Advocacy and awareness are crucial components of fighting Wolfram Syndrome. As a rare disease, there is often a lack of understanding about WS and its impact on individuals and families. It is up to advocates and awareness efforts to educate communities and push for research and resources. One way to get involved in advocacy and awareness efforts is by joining WS organizations. These groups advocate for research funding, provide support to individuals and families affected by WS, and promote awareness of the disease. Some of these organizations include the Snow Foundation and the US Wolfram Syndrome Association. Another way to get involved is by attending events and conferences related to WS. These events provide opportunities to network with other individuals and families affected by WS, meet researchers and medical professionals, and learn about new advancements in WS research and treatment. Advocacy and awareness efforts can also take place on a local level. Educating your community about WS can increase understanding and generate support. Hosting fundraisers, walks, and other events can raise funds for research and provide opportunities for increased awareness. It is important to remember that every effort, no matter how small, makes a difference in the fight against Wolfram Syndrome. By coming together and advocating for those affected by WS, we can make a lasting impact on this disease and the lives it affects. Let's continue to spread awareness and advocate for those impacted by Wolfram Syndrome.

www.ingramcontent.com/pod-product-compliance
Lightning Source LLC
Chambersburg PA
CBHW072340270726
48659CB00022B/2102